Addiction and Response

STORIES OF ADDICTION – FAILURE AND REDEMPTION

ALFRED BROCK

Story 1 - Action and Response

A short story about deadly circumstantial choices

It started simply.

Catherine hurt her ankle.

She went to the Emergency Room after waiting two days. She didn't have money to go in the first place and didn't have a regular doctor. The pain became so bad, however, that she decided to listen to her mother and go to the Emergency Room.

She left her two children with her mother and her friend, Alice, drove her over to the Emergency Room. Alice was out of work because the local Sears had closed. She used to be cashier there but the corporate structure was failing or something, she could never understand what was going on higher up at the company. It didn't matter anymore. She was out of work.

Catherine signed herself in and went through the insurance questions with the nurse at the desk. It took a long time because the nurse was distracted by other work, a telephone and the security guard kept talking to her and making jokes. Every few minutes he jiggled his gun in his holster like he was nervous. It made Catherine nervous too.

Alice was making motions like she was going to say something so Catherine asked her to go get her a drink and wait for her in the seating area. She wanted to say something too about her treatment but knew from experience that if she complained it would just make things worse or take longer to get through this. She was able to use the public insurance she had gotten after her husband left her and the nurse seemed satisfied with the answers to her questions. She was given a plastic bracelet and told to go wait in the seating area.

Catherine joined Alice and they looked through the magazines that were strewn in the area. One couple came in with three children. The father wandered around aimlessly while the mother tried to comfort a child she held in her arms that looked as if it were unconscious. The woman's little girl was reading and playing quietly. There was a little boy who looked unwashed and who walked about in an aggressive fashion banging on chairs and sliding the few toys in the children's section out into the walkway.

Others came in and were processed by the nurse at the desk. Some went immediately to see a doctor, two came in on stretchers, one accompanied by police officers, and they were wheeled to the back right away.

After waiting for two hours Catherine's name was called. She went into the back to be examined. A nurse came along and asked a few questions. She told Catherine that a doctor would be there to see her after she had X-rays done. Catherine was immediately taken by wheelchair to another hallway and parked in front of a door marked 'X-Ray'. There was a large radiation sticker on the door.

Catherine wished she had brought some of the magazines with her. She had to wait another hour before anyone showed up to talk to her. It was an orderly and he asked her what she was doing there. She told him she needed X-Rays and he went off to find one of the technicians. Thirty minutes later a technician showed up and moved Catherine into the X-Ray room and proceeded to take X-Rays of her ankle. It was a very painful procedure.

After this was done she was returned to the Emergency Room bay she had been in. She waited another 30 minutes and another nurse came in and went over the same information that the first nurse had gone over. After this was done it was another 20 minutes before a man in a white coat, who had been sitting ten feet away from the Emergency Room bay in front of a computer screen got up and walked over Catherine. He was holding a folder in front of his face and appeared to be reading it. He let it down a little and she could see he was finishing off a fruit bun.

Catherine was feeling a little hungry at this point.

'So, what's up?', said the man.

'I'm Doctor Caroll. I've seen your X-rays.'

Catherine explained how she had hurt her ankle.

'Why did you wait two days to come in?'

'I thought it would ease off.', she said.

'Oh, well, no harm done this time, but it could have been much worse. You sprained your ankle and it looks like you have a small blood clot there because of the aggravation. I believe it's just a heavy bruise, so you should be okay.'

A nurse made an appearance and talked to the doctor.

The doctor asked, 'Do you want something for the pain?'

'I don't know.', Catherine said.

'It will help you heal. You should stay off it for as much as you can over the next week.'

'Oh, alright, but something light, I can't be walking around in a daze.', Catherine responded.

The doctor left.

The nurse said, 'You can go home now. We are going to give you an ankle brace.'

The nurse also provided a prescription that had been signed by the doctor. It was for Ibuprofen and an Opioid mixed together. The doctor prescribed 60 days worth of pills. Two pills a day. One refill.

Catherine met with Alice in the waiting room. They stopped at the hospital pharmacy to get the drug. She then hobbled along out to the car on her crutches. Their conversation was mostly about worries concerning the cost of the visit. Alice said, 'Those crutches probably cost more than I earned in a week running the cash register in the clothing department.' Catherine took her first pill.

Alice dropped Catherine off. Catherine's mother was glad to see her. The two girls had gotten into a box of cookies and they were all hyped up. It took a little while but Catherine got them calmed down. Her mother said she would stay with her until her ankle healed.

60 days later Catherine was doing much better. She could walk around fairly well but there was a nagging pain in her ankle. She also felt vaguely uneasy whenever she skipped one of her pills. When her prescription ran out she had a brief discussion with her mother and Catherine decided to get the refill.

'It can't hurt, can it? Just to be sure.'

She went to the pharmacy where her request was fulfilled right away. Five dollar co-pay. It was much cheaper to get the drug than it was to see the doctor. That was for sure.

Over the next 60 days her interactions with her children changed. Not drastically but enough for the children to notice. Catherine was sleepy a lot of the time and would nap throughout the day. She had temporarily (she told her mother) abandoned her pursuit of a job to stay home and take care of the children.

She stayed home but her care of the children began to lag. She didn't even seem to notice the changes. She didn't, but the children did. They could ask Mommy for things when she was on her way to a nap or when she was sitting and staring at the tv and get what they wanted. Their behavior changed in school.

Their behavioral change in school was enough for a teacher to notice but nothing was done because there were so many children in the class that the changes that could have foretold a problem were lost in the daily shuffle of just getting things done and taking tests.

Catherine's mother didn't notice much of a difference but she was concerned that Catherine had seemed to have abandoned her job search. She was afraid Catherine would lose the house she was renting. She loved Catherine and the girls but Catherine's father was bedridden and money was tight. She couldn't imagine having Catherine move back in and bring the two girls with her.

After the second bottle of pills was done Catherine was okay at first. Over the course of the next three days, however, she became irritable, sick to her stomach and suffered the chills. Her mother had to come and stay a couple of days to help out. She told Catherine she must have the flu and did everything she could imagine that would help. Catherine refused to go to the doctor. The bills for her ankle had been extraordinary. They were going to cause hardship in her home. She was very upset.

Alice came over that weekend and as they were talking Catherine complained about how the pain in her ankle never seemed to have actually gone away. Catherine said she had some pills in her bag she had been prescribed for her surgery after her child was born and offered one to Catherine. Catherine wasn't sure at first, but with the kids running around shrieking, her mother hovering and Alice's kind face, she reached out and took the pill.

It was an unbuffered opioid.

Alice had been taking them for some time. She seemed unfazed by them. Of course, that was to anyone who had met Alice after she had started taking them. Prior to that she had been a vivacious and bubbly woman. She was a voracious reader and a hard worker. After her son was born she ended up being prescribed a set of medicines that she had eventually stopped having to take but continued to request to have her opioid pain medication rewritten.

She didn't feel comfortable without it she told the doctor. The doctor readily wrote the prescription He had a very nice relationship with his pharmaceutical distributor and from what the salesman had told him this was the best course of action against pain that there was. So triumphed advertising over 10 years of medical study.

Compassion had left the medical establishment a long time ago.

Alice bobbled along.

She gave the pill to Catherine out of friendship and love. The very next day Catherine asked for another one. Her plea was so plain and contrite that Alice knew it was the right thing to do to help her. She ended up giving her what was left in her bottle until Catherine could get a prescription.

Alice introduced Catherine to her doctor who took her insurance and assured her he would take care of her. He prescribed the exact same drug Alice was taking because of a combination of what Catherine had described to him as the failure of the pain medication she had been taking and because she asked for it specifically. Doctor Calhoun believed in working with his patients and making them part of their own care.

Catherine's medical bills, which she had been handling with her welfare checks began to mount up.

After a year of this it was clear to Catherine's mother that Catherine wasn't going to get a job. She had taken to drinking, first on the weekends with friends, and then in the evenings during the week. Her mother couldn't figure out where she was getting the money to cover her bills. It was a combination between selling some of the pills she got from the doctor and letting the others slip.

As time went on Catherine and her daughters were getting close to being evicted.

Catherine, in the meantime, had gone from relying on the expensive pills to self-medicating. She had found alternative pills that her new friends could supply her with in a trade and had even begun self-medicating with heroin and other powdered opioids. She ate it, snorted but refused to inject it because, she told Alice, that would make her an addict.

During this time Alice had allowed herself to be carried along into Catherine's new circle of friends. They began doing drugs together. The children were left with either Catherine's mother or Alice's mother. Sometimes they were left at home alone.

Cindy, the youngest at 6 years old, had gotten into Catherine's pills and nearly died. Luckily Alice's mother took the girl to the Emergency Room and had her stomach pumped. A social worker got in touch with Alice's mother at the hospital and took down all the information she was supposed to but never followed up.

Two months later at Catherine's house Alice's son, Douglas, got into a drawer that contained some drugs that Catherine was holding for her dealer. Catherine, had, by this time, moved on to injecting heroin and took on the mantle of addict proudly. Her vocabulary changed. She claimed that heroin was her first love. It was like loving Satan but being afraid of getting burned. Her behavior became more erratic.

The package that Douglas got into contained medical grade Fentanyl strips. The boy had opened a few and thinking they were stickers and decided to put them on his face. He put one on his cheek and by the time he had reached into the package to take another one out the 7 year old boy was dead.

Two weeks later Catherine overdosed in the bathroom of a bar after injecting heroin.

Alice was hospitalized for eight months. She resolved to never use drugs again. The night she went home she consumed two pills which contained fentanyl and she died.

Catherine's daughters were given over to her mother to raise.

The local hospital formed a pain committee to deal with the rise in overdose cases in their area. They were compelled to do this when State and Federal Law compelled them to or they would risk losing their tax exempt status and other benefits.

The committee had a rocky start. The head of the committee owned the pain clinic in the town. The first meetings were difficult as only an employee of the pain clinic was allowed to speak. The phone system didn't work so professionals off site could not attend. The committee decided to address the spike in opioid deaths by a combination of comfort dogs, aromatherapy and music.

Story 2 - Combustion

Corrinthia was a woman who had a set schedule. She got up in the morning every day and brushed her hair, her teeth and took a shower. She was 25 years old and still living at home with her parents. She had lost her way when she was 21. During her high school years she was a moderate student. She passed all her classes. Did not care to excel. She hung around with her friends and went with the flow.

She began drinking beer and smoking marijuana when she was 17. A little late for her neighborhood. She made up for it over time. When she turned 21 she had been in college and working on finishing her second year. She was relatively happy. When Corrinthia started dating Jack she wasn't aware of his more eccentric personal habits. They went out together and visited friends. She had even introduced him to her parents.

It was shortly after that that he introduced her to heroin and other opioids. They started snorting the drug and progressed quickly on to using it intravenously. Corrinthia, herself, never became deeply addicted, at that time, to heroin but Jack did. A year after Jack was introduced to her parents they were attending his funeral.

From then on her interaction with drugs had swung back and forth. She was in and out of rehab clinics and split her time between visiting doctors for care and trying them to get them to help her falsify prescriptions. Some of them did. One of them proposed to her that she help him get others to come see him for prescriptions. She did this for two years and the doctor grew rich. One day she went to the office to get a prescription and introduce a new addict to him and the office was closed up. She never knew if he was arrested, died or just moved on.

She remained with her parents.

Time went on.

She had become friendly with one other woman who had similar difficulties. She was a little older at 32 and had two children. What they had in common was little more than the drugs that they took together. This wasn't clear to either of them so deeply were they lost in their use and addiction.

The other woman's name was Wanda. She had been pretty before she got involved with drugs. She had two children, a girl, 7 years old, and a boy of 3. Their father had been in and out of jail over a period of ten years for minor crimes and was finally put in prison for 25 years after he stole a car and was caught with it carrying a large amount of heroin and cocaine.

His defense to the judge had been, 'I'm sorry, can I go to rehab?'

The judge replied, 'I'm sorry, too late for that, fella'. Next!'

Wanda had cried for two days. Her mother had to come to the house to feed the children. She almost lost them at that time because her mother was going to call protective services. Her mother thought better of this and decided to leave well enough alone. The scare associated with her husband's incarceration seemed to almost scare Wanda straight.

That state of mind lasted all of two days. Wanda was back out on the street looking for heroin and neglecting her children in the evening. It was a wonder neither one of them, or both, were injured or died during this period.

That's when Wanda had come across Corrinthia. Corrinthia introduced her to the doctor before he disappeared. They stayed together quite a bit. Corrinthia ended up taking care of the children most of the time. Wanda's house turned into a party zone. Wanda's boyfriends were numerous. None of them lasted very long. Some were arrested and others just wandered away.

The children spent most of the time in their room except when Corrinthia took them into the back yard which wasn't often.

As time went by Wanda became more careless with whom she would bring into her life. She brought one into her life who only went by the name Joe. No one knew his real name. Corrinthia wasn't sure Joe knew his real name. At first he was good to Wanda. He seemed to have money all the time and was generous to her.

Over the course of time he became more familiar with her. Eventually he had her picking up and delivering things for him. As time further progressed he became more demanding of her and finally possessive. Even as he sent her all through the city to pick up and deliver packages and money for him he became more resentful and jealous of her.

He was a big talker but his business operations were somewhat small. At first he seemed to be doing well but it wasn't long before it seemed he was starting to get the short end of the stick. He had begun to use drugs more heavily and his drinking followed suit. He expended money just as quickly as he seemed to make it.

Wanda went merrily along. Corrinthia was happy because both Wanda and Joe gave her drugs and her duties mostly revolved around caring for the kids. After feeding them and putting them in front of the television she spent the rest of day sitting around or sleeping until she felt the urge to use drugs again.

It was a deteriorating situation.

One day Joe came home in a rage. One of his contacts had been arrested and somehow Corrinthia's name had come up. Joe had decided that Corrinthia had something to do with the arrest and began harassing her as soon as he saw her.

Always eager to play the big man he provided some drugs to Corrinthia, who, even though Joe seemed ready to attack her, was more than happy to take them. As the fight between Joe and Wanda began, Wanda, also, gave some drugs to Corrinthia. Corrinthia, at this point, was very happy with her circumstance. The children were alternately watching the violence on television and the violence being carried out in their living room.

Corrinthia became more and more inebriated. She could feel her breath slowing. She had no intention of moving. The scenes playing out before her seemed farther and farther away.

The fight between the two stoned gladiators continued on through the afternoon. At dinnertime Wanda made some attempt at cooking and provided macaroni and cheese and beans to the kids. The children remained in front of the television and generally seemed to ignore the shouting and banging going on behind them.

Corrinthia continued to sink into her stupor.

It was sometime around 8 o'clock when Joe and Wanda came to blows. They struck out at each other, sometimes successfully, and more often than not, unsuccessfully. Their continued torrent of verbal abuse strayed in and out of coherence. In a dark comic mix Wanda and Joe both walked out of the house on each other twice. It was during the last of these lulls that the children climbed up on the couch together.

Corrinthia leaned back in her recliner and was watching the television with one eye. The other eye half closed. Wanda had then begun Joe to get out. She repeatedly shouted, 'Just get out'. He would shout back, 'Where do expect me to go?'

To which Wanda would respond, 'Back where you came from.'

At about 8:30 PM Joe stormed back into the house. He stood in front of Wanda who was sitting in a chair opposite Corrinthia. He demanded she tell him what she had been doing all day. She said, 'I was arguing with you. Get out!'

Joe said, 'You're really burning me up! I'm gonna' burn you up!'

'Just try it, you creep!', Wanda called out.

From his pocket Joe removed a can of lighter fluid. In a moment he had popped the top open. He squirted it all over Wanda who was still yelling at him and now surprised that she was wet.

She yelled at him, 'What do you think you're doing?'

At which point Joe pulled out a lighter and reached over and ignited the liquid.

Corrinthia watched in a slow realization of horror that her friend had just been lit on fire.

The children glanced over and were looking on as well as they played with their toys.

'That'll show ya'!', yelled Joe as he stomped out of the house.

The flames had started out flickering but slowly increased. Wanda started to cry out and her voice slowly escalated into howls and shrieks the kind of which Corrinthia had never heard in her life.

The flames increased in brightness and still Corrinthia sat staring at the spectacle before her. She did not reach out to the children. She did nothing.

Wanda ran to the shower screaming, 'Help, help, me!'. She succeeded igniting the shower curtain as she turned the water on. Her hair caught on fire and her clothes were ablaze and she was screaming as she threw herself in the shower. She sank down into the tub and it just because she accidently pressed her foot on the drain plug that water began accumulate and allowed her to put the fire out and stop her body from burning.

She lay in the tub moaning and crying for over two hours before Corrinthia could get out of her chair. It was another half hour before she called the police as Corrinthia made a bizarre attempt to hide any evidence of drug use. She never bothered to see to the children who ended up asleep on the couch.

They were there when the police arrived. A social services worker was called. Wanda was taken to the hospital where she began a long period of burn therapy.

Joe returned the next day and the neighbors told him the police were looking for him. He quickly made off. He was picked up three months later in another city for possession. He was released on bond and never seen again.

She was happy to attend the training. Kate had heard about it from a friend and she was amazed at what she had been told. By using Narcan she might be able to save a life. She might be able to save the life of her friend – maybe even her boyfriend.

Kate's boyfriend, Roger, had been using heroin for about two years. She was so sorry that he used the drug. She blamed herself for his using the drug. She blamed herself for his starting to use the drug in the first place.

She was sure it was her fault because Roger told her it was her fault. He told her nearly every single day. She wasn't one to give up and wanted to fight for Roger's life, even if he wasn't interested in it.

She decided to learn all she could about drug addiction and she did. She took classes at the local community college and worked as a volunteer at the local hospital. She was also a volunteer at the local drug court. Not the one that Roger had been sent through, but another one, in the next town of Velma. She spent a lot of time in Velma and had made many friends there. One woman in particular had become very close to her.

Susan was the one who told Kate about Narcan. Susan was wise in the ways of the world and realized that Kate's predicament was a little more than the dangers posed by Roger's drug use. Susan realized that Kate was trapped in an abusive relationship. She gently urged Kate to get away from Roger but stopped short of overtly condemning Roger. Kate was lost in her relationship and it was far beyond Susan's ability to break it up.

She did help Kate in every way she could, however, and Kate responded. Over time Susan was sure, that if the relationship didn't turn to outright violent abuse or Kate was exposed to fentanyl or killed or hurt in collateral violence over drugs or money that the relationship would probably break up on its own.

Roger didn't seem like the kind of guy who would stick around long.

He had shown up Blossom, Georgia, just a couple of months before meeting Kate. He had passed out in one of the aisles in the dollar store where Kate worked. She had immediately begun taking care of him. She even shielded him from the police officer that showed up looking for him that day. She had Roger sitting in the back with an ice pack on his head when the officer came in asking questions.

She had deferred telling the officer that the man he was looking for was sitting in the storeroom watching the flickering tv and cooling his head. She had even placed a band aid on a small cut he had on his forehead.

Kate was a kind and forgiving person. She took to Roger immediately who had all the charm and skills of a con artist. He convinced her he was a down on his luck salesman and was just looking for a big break. He said he was working on a million dollar deal and was getting everything set up to pull it off. She believed him but not really. Kate was kind but not stupid. She just didn't pay attention when his stories of his grandiose schemes change. She did pay attention, however, whenever he passed out from drug use. She would swing into action like Florence Nightingale and care for him and bind his wounds.

One thing she found she could not do was to wake him up all the time. Sometimes she just could not. His shallow breathing would send her into a panic. She didn't know what to do. That is when she started to study.

Her studies on behalf of Roger led Kate to do good things for many other people. It turned out that her amiable manner and conversational style were good tools to have in the medical field and she ended up working towards becoming a practical nurse. She started the courses just six months after meeting Roger and she only had six months more to go.

Kate's parents were confused and excited. They had known their girl was smart but she had never seemed to apply herself. They were ecstatic that she was attending school and doing well. They were confused by Kate's relationship with Roger. He seemed a nice enough fellow when they first met him but it wasn't long before they notice something was wrong. Roger didn't work, first of all. He also kept odd hours. Sometimes he would be gone all night and at other times would be gone for days at a time.

He might return looking well or he might return looking like he had been in hell. He would be covered with bruises, his clothes torn and blood all around. They saw all this because Kate still lived at home and Roger had come to live with her in their house.

They didn't know what to do but were afraid to be forceful in their condemnation of Roger because they didn't want to lose contact with their daughter and accidently push her into the world she was so closely skating near.

Susan told Kate about Narcan and the two of them went to a local training.

Narcan is a drug that can be used when a person is suspected of an opioid overdose. It must be performed by someone other than the patient. Kate and Sue went to a local club where alcoholics met to attend the meeting. The manager of the Club, Ben, was keenly interested in helping the addicts he knew lived all around the area. He also knew Roger and suspected that he was not only an addict but one of the local dealers who was causing all the trouble.

During their training they were instructed to read the Instructions for Use at the time they receive the prescription for Narcan Nasal Spray. They were clearly told to following instructions

They were to administer Narcan Nasal Spray as quickly as possible because prolonged respiratory depression may result in damage to the central nervous system or death.

Kate knew that the duration of action of most opioids exceeds that of naloxone hydrochloride and the suspected opioid overdose may occur outside of supervised medical settings, seek immediate emergency medical assistance, keep the patient under continued surveillance until emergency personnel arrive, and administer repeated doses of Narcan Nasal Spray, as necessary. She became aware that she needed to always seek emergency medical assistance in the event of a suspected, potentially life-threatening opioid emergency after administration of the first dose of Narcan Nasal Spray.

What was meant by the fact that "duration of action of most opioids exceeds that of naloxone hydrochloride and the suspected opioid overdose may occur outside of supervised medical settings" was that if someone was overdosing on an opioid and Narcan was administered as the antidote, then the person who had just suffered the overdose needed to get to the hospital or other official medical care because the Narcan reverses the effects but doesn't last as long in the bloodstream as the opioids do. Without further care the person that had been revived might lapse back into overdose and die or become physically or mentally incapacitated for the rest of their life.

Kate paid close attention when she was told that additional doses of Narcan Nasal Spray may be required until emergency medical assistance becomes available. The prescription she was given came with two doses. She became familiar with the ingredients right away.

The other things they learned included that they should not attempt to reuse Narcan Nasal Spray. Each Narcan Nasal Spray contains a single dose of naloxone and cannot be reused. The instructor made it clear that though were two doses in the package there was only one dose in each container.

The instructor told them that they may need to re-administer Narcan Nasal Spray, using a new nasal spray, every 2 to 3 minutes if the patient does not respond or responds and then relapses into respiratory depression.

One of the women at the training burst into tears. Her husband held her up. She kept asking him, 'Why is he doing this? Why is he making us do something like this? He's poisoning himself!'.

The instructor gave everyone a break and they cared for the woman who regained her composure after a short time.

The students were shown how to administer Narcan Nasal Spray in alternate nostrils with each dose and to administer Narcan Nasal Spray according to the printed instructions on the device label and the Instructions for Use.

Kate and Susan learned that it is very important to place the patient in the supine position and before administration make sure the device nozzle is inserted in either nostril of the patient or it would just spray all over the place. They were shown how to provide support to the back of the neck to allow the neck to tilt back. The woman who had cried out again became hysterical saying she wasn't strong enough to do that and her husband assured her, with help from the instructor, that they would get a pillow to help in case anything happened.

It turned out that the person they were concerned about was their son. The boy was 21 years old and had been using heroin for about a year. He had already had three overdoses in the house, each time rescued by local Emergency Medical Technicians. This training was the result of encouragement from the family's pastor. Truth be told he wished his entire congregation would go because they had already lost three parishioners within two years. He knew, unfortunately, that if they couldn't save their son they might be able to save someone else. The pastor was there that evening also.

He was only pastor in the town that responded in any way to the announcement of the training. He was very disappointed in his clerical co-workers of other faiths and religions but he could only do what he could. He could only do what God called him to do.

Everyone was relieved when they all got a turn to press on the device plunger firmly and administer a dose of life saving liquid to the poisoned dummy they were using as a stand-in for an overdosing human being.

After administering the dose the next step is to turn the person on their side, so that, if they should vomit they will not block their airway and choke to death while waiting for the ambulance.

After everyone had a try they were all given a sample. They spent a short time afterward eating cookies, drinking juice and talking. Finally, they all went home.

It was about two weeks later that Roger had a problem. He had left town a week after Kate had attended her training. She encouraged him to carry Narcan but he said he didn't need it. She said he might be able to help someone else.

He asked her, 'Who do you think I am? What do I care about someone else for? They should be able to take care of themselves like I do.'

This came as no surprise to Kate. She just didn't pay attention to it.

When Roger came back he looked in a bad way. He looked as if he had been beaten and he was clearly nearly out of his mind with drug use. He had brought back yet another car with him. This one had Mississippi plates. He insisted that Kate's parents stay away from it and to allow him to park it in the garage with the door shut.

After he had been back for a week he was looking a little better but his behavior was erratic. He was under the influence of drugs most of the time and slept a lot.

The next Saturday evening Susan came to visit Kate. Kate's parents liked Susan. They all had dinner together and sat down to watch a movie. Roger went out and returned after an hour. He was looking ill.

He sat down in one of the chairs and began to speak loudly. He used abusive language to everyone present. Kate told him he needed to stop. At which point he leapt out of his chair and began screaming. He was flailing his hands in the air. Kate's parents had never seen him like this. They began to be afraid. Susan was afraid that he would attack Kate right in front of them. She tried to formulate a plan but had been caught off guard.

Then Roger began to wretch. He vomited on the floor and fell over on his side. Kate's parents and Susan looked on in disbelief.

Kate calmly stood up, went to the bathroom, opened the medicine cabinet and brought back the Narcan. She administered the drug just as she had been shown. She called for medical help just as she had learned. She administered the drug again.

Nothing happened. Roger had stopped breathing.

Kate administered Narcan again.

No change.

She administered it again.

Nothing.

Susan said, 'That's enough, Kate. You've done enough.'

Kate said, 'I know.'

The doorbell rang. Susan opened it and the Emergency Medical Technicians came in. There were two of them. They went to work quickly and efficiently. Kate calmly answered all their questions.

Eventually one of the technicians said, 'I'm sorry, Miss. He's dead.'

Kate said, 'I know, but why? I gave him Narcan.'

The medic said, 'I see that. You did well, but, he was on more than opioids. It looks like he was using methamphetamine as well and possibly cocaine. We'll have to test. From what happened here it seems like his heart just exploded.'

Kate said, 'Okay. That makes sense. You can take him away.'

After Roger's body was removed Kate cleaned up the mess.

Six months later she received her Practical Nursing license and started classed become a Registered Nurse.

Story 4 – Finding

Lori was a mother. She was a normal mother for 18 years. She gave birth, took her son to church enrolled him in school, provided him with birthday parties, fed him, clothed him, went to school to talk with his teachers, helped him with minor problems as we progressed into young adulthood and then things changed.

Sometime during the last two years of his high school career young James had become acquainted with the drugs. He started drinking beer at parties and out in parks and progressed to smoking marijuana. The neighborhood and area in which James and his parents lived was fairly well off. There was no unemployment problem. Most of the people in the area had reasonably good jobs in manufacturing and other industries. The community was mixed between white collar and blue collar workers.

The normal expectation by the parents for the children in the area was to at least finish high school. Many targeted college as the next step in their educational career but not all.

What the children had was a little spending money. The parents gave them the money freely and there was generally very little accounting of where it went. The general expectations were that they kids would spend it on cheeseburgers, movies, electronic games and sports events. The reality was that there weren't many places to get a cheeseburger. The kids could choose between three McDonald's in the area or one Taco Bell if they were feeling adventurous. As for movies there were two megatheaters. One was in a mall and the other by itself in a gargantuan strip mall next to Home Depot on the edge of town. Both of them charged a lot for their tickets and snacks which were unhealthy anyway. As for electronic games the kids could go to the local arcade in the mall where about a quarter of the games at any given time were not working or they could buy the games for exorbitant prices and bring them home where their parents would complain they played them too much. Finally there was sports events – it turned out that it was after sports events that James had picked up the habit of drinking beer and later smoking marijuana.

Through his sports contacts he also was exposed to pill form pain medication, powered opioids and eventually heroin.

He was addicted to opioids by the middle of his senior year and by the time he graduated from high school he had also 'graduated' to using heroin intravenously – that is, he was injecting heroin into his bloodstream with a needle.

He became a classic addict.

It was the summer after he graduated from high school that he had first serious brush with the law. His parents intervened and they went through an entire process of 'getting clean', meeting with 'peer coaches' and learning about halfway houses. This entire set of experiences put a chill into Lori's marriage and his husband Richard asked for a divorce later that year. They parted amicably.

Lori became saddled with James. It didn't seem that way at the time but he became more and more of a burden as time went on. He asked for money, lived at the house and went through several jobs. He didn't stay long wherever he worked and when not working he had become adept at finding public assistance for food and even paying for lodging – money he never turned over to his mother.

His entire presentation to his mother was a lie. She could see through it sometimes but being busy with her own life and honestly being concerned with James and believing him and in him she missed many of the clues, or ignored them, that would have indicated James was not doing well at all.

He moved on from just using drugs to holding them for the hoodlums he bought them from. He was relatively intelligent and used his cunning and knowledge to further his way with the dealers. It wasn't long before he was dealing himself and helping to move the drugs through the area.

He strayed away from contact with his mother. She didn't hear from him even though he lived close by.

At one point he was cornered and arrested. The police offered him a chance to avoid long term prison by cooperating with them. He decided to go with this and ended up playing a part in getting one of the larger dealers in the area arrested.

He was pleasantly surprised after all this was done to be approached by another dealer who happened to take over from the guy who was imprisoned. The new dealer offered James an even more lucrative position in his organization. He kept with this for five years and by the time he had reached the age of 26 he had his own home, a car and was living well in the same neighborhood his parents had raised him in.

During all this time he was trafficking marijuana, illicit prescpription opioids, heroin and occasionally cocaine.

Just before he turned 27 he was arrested again.

Again his testimony and information helped to convict other dealers and users.

The result of this incarceration, however, was different. All of his possessions were confiscated. His car, his house, cash, all his goods and his boat which had become his pride and joy.

When released from prison about three months later he was destitute. He had no money, no food and no prospects.

It wasn't long before he began practicing the only craft he know – drug dealing. He was not trusted anymore, however, and he was forced to small deals. He started using heavily so anything he made he ended up consuming. This was when he came back into Lori's life.

He asked for a place to live.

She refused.

He asked for money.

She refused.

He began to confide in her telling her he had taken to dealing in order to support his habit.

She told him that if he had enough money to buy drugs he had enough money to buy food. She told him if he had enough gumption to deal drugs he had the ability to find a place to live.

He then began a periodic process of coming back to her every couple of days, either by stopping by or calling her, and asking for help.

Lori came to her wits end and asked her friend Jody what to do.

Lori told Jody that James had been getting deeply involved in drugs over the past year and according to him had been injecting heroin and methamphetamine.

Jody was shocked by the whole thing. She had been friends with Lori a long time. She was aware of the history with James. What shocked her was James' insistence and his constant, sudden, contact with his estranged mother.

Jody tried to communicate her unease to Lori but was unsuccessful in putting it into words.

One day James showed up at Lori's house while Jody was there.

He even asked Jody for help.

Jody was, at first, unable to articulate her response.

She finally came up with a few words and followed closely those things that Lori had said. She wasn't going to give him any money or help and he should take care of himself.

At this point he became verbally abusive to Jody and asked her why she was always hanging around with his mother. He accused her of turning his mother against him. His tirade grew in ferocity as he went on. Jody told him that she wasn't going to take that from him.

Lori told him to stop as well but he didn't listen. He went from asking for money to demanding it. His mother told him if he didn't leave she was going to call the police.

He became infuriated at this point and said he would never leave. His mother then went to the phone and began to dial 9-1-1 at which point James ran out of the house.

He had only a few dollars in his pocket. He made his way to a drug house he knew in the neighborhood which was owned by the man who took the mantle of local drug dealer from him after James had been arrested the last time.

James was successful in getting drugs from the man. He had to pay over what was left in his pockets and promise to never return. The dealer told him the house had been watched and having James show up was bad for business all around.

James took the drugs and went to a friend's house. They went into the basement of the home where his friend Randall lived with his own parents. James took the drugs he had bought, which were several doses, and began to consume them. After a while Randall asked James to leave because his parents were coming home. He had been barely successful in getting them to believe he was not using drugs but having James there would tip his hand.

James got Randall to allow him to stay by giving him a dose of heroin.

Randall set James up in a small guest bedroom in the basement and told him to be quiet.

James laid down on the bed and injected heroin. He lay quietly for a while and then followed that with an injection of methamphetamine and another dose of heroin.

While Randall was upstairs with his parents having dinner Randall explained to them his plan for getting a new job the following week. They suspected he was on drugs but said nothing. Their own plans were wrapped up in how they could get help for Randall. They were split as a couple between doing all they could to help him and throwing him out of the house.

The only reason they hadn't thrown him out yet was that he seemed to be rather subdued. He didn't make that much trouble and they believed they had time to help him out before something bad happened.

The next morning Randall's father discovered James' body.

Story 5 – Making a Profit

Bill leaned back in his chair.

The numbers didn't add up.

Bill liked his chair.

If the numbers were correct, and he was sure they were, they weren't going to hit their goals.

Bill felt comfortable in the heavy leather upholstery.

The shareholders were going to hit the roof.

Bill liked to just look at the chair but he enjoyed sitting in it even more. It was an overstuffed, brown, leather chair fixed with brass fastenings. It had two large arm holders and big casters on the floor so he could roll around when he felt like it. He didn't feel like it right at that moment.

He looked at the computer screen again.

Well, no other way around it. He'd have to do something different if he was going to keep the chair. He really liked that chair.

Bill Reynolds had been in the rehab business for over 20 years. He had been expecting to retire during his next go-round but according to what he was looking at now that wasn't going to happen. At least not the way he had planned it.

Bill was a conscientious worker. He had worked hard to become the director of the 'Fine Hills Rehabilitation Clinic'. Bill started out as a good student at a good high school. He went on to a fine college where he played on the tennis team. He considered going professional but the time and effort weren't something he wanted to expend. He wanted something else out of life.

While he was looking for that something else he found drugs. As it was his tennis career and academic career wrapped up about the same time as his drug use started to cycle up. He obtained his sports honors and academic credentials and so was able to find a reasonably good paying job.

He spent most of his money on 'recreational' drugs, however. He became an advocate for legalizing marijuana. He started a 'Medicinal Marijuana' shop that was little more than a pot shop. The small town he had set up in tolerated him until he decided to add vaping equipment. They busted him for selling rolling paper and confiscated all his goods and the shop. He had had to declare bankruptcy.

He almost stopped using drugs at that time but circumstances pushed him on to using more. He enjoyed bankruptcy and was able to use the laws to start up a small restaurant which he also ran into the ground but more for traditional reasons because restaurants are hard businesses to start up.

He ended up destitute and homeless. He had a criminal record and was put into a rehabilitation program. It was a peculiarity of his situation, life choices, connection and family that his insurance covered the expenses of his care and treatment and the facility he went to. Unlike most of the other 'inmates', as he called them, he paid attention to the bills that were being generated and the amounts being paid out.

He watched, at first with sadness and sorrow, as parents, families and friends came to visit some of his compatriots. He was shocked to learn how much they paid out of their pockets for the treatment he was getting through insurance. Those without insurance seemed to pay even more than he did. There were tales of them showing up and paying $40,000, $60,000 and more for a short stay. Later his emotional concern for their loss turned to more personal interest.

As he leaned even further back in his leather 'King Chair' as he called it, he remembered how one night he had sat down in the common room with a pencil and pad and instead of doodling as he normally did he began doing the math to figure out how much money the facility was taking in.

He shook his head in wonder as he stared at the bottom line.

What a gold mine!

If anything caused him to work towards escaping the scourge of drugs it was the profit margin.

He stopped thinking about getting illicit drugs and began to think of ways of how to get out of the facility. He learned what he needed to do – it turned out they had clearly told him when he arrived – and he followed all of their directions to the 'T'.

The 'Cure' cost quite a bit but it did work – if the person were dedicated and followed all the instructions and duties associated with it. Bill learned that most of the problems associated with cost overruns for care were due to several factors, that, thankfully, weren't affecting him.

The first pitfall to those shelling out the money for the drug cure was the cooperation of the person being treated. At first Bill had thought most of the people in the facility were there because they were out of control and couldn't help themselves. It was amazing to him, then, to discover, that a sizeable number of them were there merely pretending to go along with the treatment. Their main goal was not to 'get better' and 'recover' but to get out of the place and use drugs again.

That aspect of the emotional pain being exhibited by the visitors to the 'inmates' that were living their life that way was initially disturbing to Bill. He was appalled at their cruelty to their loved ones and amazed at the credulity of those who continued to pay.

There was, of course, extenuating circumstances that allowed this to happen. First of all – the 'inmates', 'patients' or 'addicts', to use different names for them, had a very sophisticated system for duping the system. They helped each other. They were clever. They were deceitful. It was like watching a den of thieves, thought Bill at the time, the only thing wrong with the picture was that the thieves were stealing from themselves.

Along with the general population of people being served there were the few like Bill, who woke up and wanted out forever. There was also a sliver of the population, who, once the drugs were removed as a barrier, exhibited all the behaviors of people with mental illness. Some of them were helped at that time. Others could not or would not be helped and continued on through the cycle of addiction and recovery along with the rest.

Within six months of exiting the facility Bill had a half-way house set up. He had started a non-profit, bought the house, furnished it and populated it. He had an income. With that income he worked to open other 'recovery' locations which housed people fresh out of some rehabilitation facility or jail. He kept his facilities separate but others in his business mixed them together. The result of mixing them together led to a high rate of recidivism – that is the drug users went back to using drugs and the criminals went back to their criminal activities. The difference, a lot of the time was that the drug addicts and the criminals combined their life experiences and turned into drug addicted criminals.

After a year and a half of running the business successfully he was able to buy into a larger organization that ran a larger facility. Within five years he was the director and within ten he had sold it at a hefty profit to investors.

He then started another facility and built it into a thriving business. Not only were there lots of people for him to work with there was plenty of return business. They just kept coming back. Even after all this time he was still amazed at what parents would do to pay him to take care of their kids for a couple of months. Some would remortgage or even sell their homes. They would liquidate stock, empty bank accounts and take wild loans. They would do this even after he told them the realities of the situation and what to expect.

It would have been heartbreaking but Bill still got a thrill every time they handed over a check.

The work was generally pleasant. He kept out of the wards and hardly the patients anymore. He had done a good business starting smaller recovery houses and then selling them to investors. He had dabbled in the industry in Florida but had been disgusted by the mortality rate and, he had to admit, he was scared off by the investigations coming down the pike.

The immediate problem he had now was that the numbers weren't panning out.

They had been doing a brisk business and with the opioid epidemic getting worse every year it looked like the sky was the limit in the drug rehabilitation business. The better insurance coverage companies were paying regularly and Bill's clinic had very few declinations when covered patients checked in. Of course, if they weren't covered and could pay on their own the money was no problem. Bill had to keep a tight lid on his intake personnel because sometimes they might get a little aggressive. It was important keep the patient the focus of the situation and not the ability of the people to pay.

To put it more plainly – it hurt business to be obvious about how it was a business.

Bill was doing well. He had set himself up well. It was time to get out and Bill would do that well as well. He would see to it.

He decided two months prior he would sell the facility but he couldn't get a buyer right now. He had priced it right and set up everything the way he was supposed to but the market was saturated, even though it was still lucrative. All around him detox and rehab center owners historically resorted to overly aggressive marketing tactics to pick the short-term money and flip the properties to private equity buyers who would repeat the process.

In that cycle the level of care at a facility would spiral downward until in the end it would resemble little more than a stopping place on the way to the streets after getting out of jail or running out of money to pay at the clinic.

Lately, however, that hadn't been profitable for the 'operators', of which Bill was one, but in his case he had the good sense to make quality pay. He was being impacted by the current market nonetheless. At the fringe of his thinking were the plans and moves that the unscrupulous operators would pull but he just didn't have the stomach for the body count that ultimately started to accumulate at the end of a facility's cycle. There was just no accounting for that. It was as vicious and brutal as the drug business it was supposed to help counter.

The strategy to exploit the rehabilitation properties had been successful for decades. Some of the investing groups were legitimate investment groups, retirement plans and foreign investors. Many of them foolishly did not know where their money was going to. Some of them clearly did and didn't care.

As health insurance coverage costs and ways to pay for them changed along with laws to ensure that drug addiction therapy was more stringently overseen the impact on the industry had become clear. Rather than imposing more oversight, however, the regulations had not actually been applied. They weren't being practiced. The regulations had simply melted away. Along with the levels of care being impacted the insurers were no longer paying as they once had. The past two months had seen a flurry of cancellations and ending business for the clinic. It was made clear that it wasn't due to the services provided by Bill's clinic – it was merely the fact that because they weren't being forced to pay the insurers weren't going to.

It looked like the lawsuits against the drug manufacturers were going to be a deciding factor in the future but Bill couldn't wait that long. It could be twenty or thirty years before the drew any blood out that turnip. He had gotten into the business for the long haul but not that long.

There was also the fact that even though the pharmaceutical companies had caused the opioid epidemic if they were all run out of business that wouldn't impact the drug problems caused by cocaine, kratom, marijuana (legal or otherwise), barbituates, methamphatemines and a host of other drugs.

No, the problem the industry was facing now was liquidity.

Bill was sure he could go on pulling in enough from the families and personal savings of those he had in the clinic and those expected to come but that would not feed the growth that was necessary to keep the place afloat and make a profit for himself.

He could dedicate the rest of his life to the place but he wasn't interested in continuing to work with staffing issues. Many of the people who worked themselves into the rehabilitation industry were themselves people who had gone through the misery of drug addiction and the related diseases. Bill wasn't looking forward to living in that world forever.

He had a great reputation and so did the clinic so it would make it easer to do what he had in mind.

He had a good competitive advantage in the area and enjoyed the support of local governments and businesses willing to push their problems off onto him. He found that aspect of the business unsavory and wouldn't miss it.

He books were in order and six months out they still looked good. It was at that time he determined that an entire different level of effort would be needed to run the place profitably and he wasn't willing to do that that.

Two things had kept him from liquidating immediately.

The first one was the admissions rate. It was climbing precipitously. If he had been a different person he might have felt a twinge of guilt about walking out when the tide turned just as everyone showed up on the beach. He wasn't that type of person so he didn't think about it.

The second one was the survivability rate.

He had gone over the numbers over and over again.

There was no doubt about it.

The survivability rate of the clinic was the highest of all the facilities in the state. It had one of the highest rates in the country and might, indeed, if such things had been quantified by any responsible body, been shown to be the highest in the country.

What would happen if he stopped doing what he was doing?

He didn't know. The investors would need to get involved and find another director.

The best he could do was not do anything. He didn't know why his clinic was the best. He just knew it was about to start losing money and there was nothing he could do about it.

In an uncharacteristic move he did what he could to perpetuate the structure of the organization after he left. Nothing was binding, of course, once he did what he did he would have no further control. He would only have his money.

So – he changed the clinic into a Foundation. He transferred all funds into the Foundation which provided instructions for how the clinic was to continue operating. He notified all the principals in the organization of their new roles and duties. He notified the bank and investors. He then paid himself out as his last act as director of the clinic and turned the operation over to the general manager.

As he left the grounds another ambulance rolled in through the gates. A man and a woman in a car followed behind. They looked confused and tired.

Bill rolled his chair down the handicapped ramp and had two orderlies put it into the back of his SUV.

Bill drove home.

Story 6

Sally and the Hot Dog

She sat in front of me. She looks sad. Her name is Sally. She told me she was married. She told me she like to talk to me. I asked her where she lived. The town she mentioned was close to mine.

We were at a barbecue. Held by my friend. My wife was there too. She was talking to her friends. I had ended up sitting with Sally because I saw her alone. I had heat up my plate with hot dogs, macaroni salad, grapes and chips. I was also juggling a drink.

I sat down heavily. I almost dropped everything. Sally reached out quickly and helped me. I sat down and started to eat. I noticed she hadn't gotten anything. I asked her if she was hungry.

She said, "No."

She said she had eaten earlier. She sat quietly for 10 minutes. Then she said, "I don't even know why I came today."

I looked at her in surprise. I kept on eating. She was pretty. She seemed like a nice person. I was wondering what she meant.

I was wolfing down a hot dog and preparing to ask her what she meant and she continued.

"I don't mean to be mean. I am glad I came. I just don't know why. I've been so unhappy lately."

Now I noticed she looked plenty tired. Like she hadn't slept or slept well for a while. She clutching her bag like she was ready to run. I swallowed my hot dog and ask her if she wanted something to drink, maybe some water.

She said, 'Water would be fine.'

I got up to get her a bottle. At the table I saw my wife and she asked me if Sally was bothering me. I said, 'No.'

She told me Sally gets a little weird sometimes and she went off with one of her friends.

I brought the bottle to Sally. I began working on my second hot dog. Sally checked her phone. She put the phone back in her purse. She said to me, 'I know they think I'm weird. I'm just tired.'

I chuckled a little. I said, ' It's good to get your rest.'

Then she began, 'I just don't know what to do. I've been married for 10 years. I've got two beautiful children. My parents are supportive. I've got a pretty good job. I enjoy where I live.

My husband. He just doesn't get it. Is not working. He's living with his girlfriend. Well she might be his girlfriend or sometimes. It's crazy. She's his drug dealer.

He's living with her. I don't know what else. He thinks he can get it for free for the rest of his life. I just don't know how long that's going to last.

When he was living home he would literally stay up for days at a time. Then he would crash and sleep for what seemed like days at a time. I didn't know what to do. I threatened to throw him out. I threw him out. I took him back. Back and forth. Back and forth. Now he's gone.

I don't know what to do. Should I support him? Should I dump him? The kids don't even know him. I don't know him. I promised till death do us part. So it's like that. What do you think?'

I looked at her. I was still chewing the last part oh my second hot dog. I was looking forward to my potato salad. I thought for a moment.

I said, 'It's up to you. There are a lot of things to consider. I just met you. Your problems are monumental. I could give you the man answer and tell you exactly what I think you should do. I feel that would be wrong. I've done that a lot with my wife. It caused a lot of trouble. I try not to do that now. I don't think I should do that with you. What you've told me is that your husband is no longer in your children's life. Is that so?'

She nodded in the affirmative.

I said, 'I don't understand is continued contact with you. Maybe you are a source for money. Maybe somewhere he feels guilty. Maybe somewhere he wants to go home but it doesn't seem like that is true. The decision is yours. I will say this I believe the children need the best of everything we can give them and also the best of everything we are.'

She sat quietly and looked at her hands.

'You want a hot dog and some potato salad?'

She answered, 'Yes, please.'.

I got it for her.

Story 7

The Notary

Part 1

Rita looked down at her hands.

She sat quietly in the room. She was surrounded by sixteen other people in similar circumstances to her own and one moderator. Well, they, similar circumstances was exaggerating it a bit. They all had different circumstances. Some were poor and had been bussed over from the shelter to attend the meeting, some were single, some were married, at least two appeared to be well off, if not rich. Rather than saying they had similar circumstances, it might be more accurate to say they had something in common.

The thing they had in common was drugs. Then, again, they didn't all have problems with drugs, or at least, if you consider alcohol a drug, not all the same drugs. There were people in the room that showed the droopy eyes and sallow skin of the alcoholic, there was one woman who wore a smart pantsuit and never took off her coat – she had the jumpy and jerky moves that Rita had come to associate with cocaine use. There were four people with the yellow skin and far off eyes that bespoke opioid addiction.

The primary reason they were all there was because they had been ordered there from the drug court.

It was Rita's turn to talk. She reached into her pocket and took out a piece of paper. Printed on it were the words used in the wedding ceremony performed by notary publics in the State of Florida. The entire process was approved by the Governor. That was one of the duties the Governor enjoyed in Florida, she thought, some sort of religious leader in a society pledge to keep church and state separate.

She unfolded the paper and looked at it. She read through it quickly before she started to talk.

She read :

"Sample Wedding Ceremony

Notary states, "Dearly beloved, we are gathered here today (tonight) to join this man and this woman in (holy) matrimony."

Exchange of Vows Notary asks the man, "(his name), do you take this woman to be your wife, to live together in (holy) matrimony, to love her, to honor her, to comfort her, and to keep her in sickness and in health, forsaking all others, for as long as you both shall live?"

Man answers, "I do."

Notary asks the woman, "(her name), do you take this man to be your husband, to live together in (holy) matrimony, to love him, to honor him, to comfort him, and to keep him in sickness and in health, forsaking all others, for as long as you both shall live?"

Woman answers, "I do."

Notary states, "Repeat after me.""

Part 2

After she read it out loud she sat quietly for a moment.

She remembered what had been happening to her over the past few months.

She recalled one time while they were driving to see his parents on the other side of the state that when they had stopped at a rest area they had parked under some trees. It was a beautiful day. She was so happy to be out with him and in the country.

He was drunk, of course.

After they had pulled out of the rest area and onto the highway she had been talking about how happy she was and that they were going to see his parents.

They drove without speaking for just a few minutes. He suddenly braced his knees against the steering wheel and then grabbed her by the hair. He pulled her head back with his right hand and quickly and forcibly punched in the face with his left.

He immediately went back to driving the car.

She recalled that, after she had stopped crying, she turned to him and said, 'I'm sorry.'

She just couldn't remember why she had said that.

Later that night, after they had arrived at his parent's house, he crushed a beer can into the side of her face. She touched the scar that was still there as she looked up and gazed around the room at the other participants.

'My husband is getting ready to go to Rehab. I love him very much. When he goes away I don't want him to come back, is that wrong?'

Most of the people in the room weren't looking at her. Three of them weren't even paying attention at all. They looked like they couldn't wait to get out of the room.

The moderator asked some gentle questions and tried to steer the conversation on and past what was becoming a very tense and embarrassing situation.

One woman on the other side of the room put up her hand.

The moderator said, 'Yes, Brenda? Do you have something to say.'

Brenda said, 'It's not wrong. You can leave him if you want to. It will all be alright.'

She looked at Brenda for about twenty seconds and then shook her head very quickly up and down. Stifling a small cry she said, 'Thank you.'

Brenda replied, 'Don't mention it. It's been enough. I can tell. We can all tell.'

About thirty minutes later the meeting ended and as they were eating cookies and drinking a little coffee the moderator approached her and said, 'That went well, didn't it?'

She answered, 'Yes, it did.'

She went home and found the house empty. Her heart skipped a beat. She sat by the door with her bag packed. She was ready to return to her own parents who had invited her home.

She waited and then a car pulled up.

There were footsteps on the walkway.

He walked in the door. He was a little unsteady.

She asked, 'Are you going to Rehab? Do you want me to drive?'

He grimaced at her and said, 'No, I've decided not to go.'

He turned and followed up with, 'Get dinner ready, I'm going to take a shower.'

He left the room.

She stood up. She picked up her bag. She went out the door. She walked down the path. She got in her car. She drove off and never returned.

Story 8

Let Me Tell You My Story

Betty was looking at the mirror.

She didn't know what to do.

She turned back to her computer screen. She 'Liked' a picture of a kitten her friend in Alabama posted.

She turned her head to the television and watched the images flicker across the screen. A fire truck. A newscaster. Some rain. She turned back to the computer screen.

She wrote slowly into the comment section, 'I'm an alcoholic.'

'I just came to that conclusion. There can be no other. I drink all the time. I drink in the morning, I drink in the afternoon, I drink at night. I drink on the weekend. I drink during the week.'

'It's a problem. I don't want to do this anymore. I feel so alone.'

Her fingers hovered above the keyboard. Should she press 'Send'?

It had been a long time coming, she realized. Betty, 38 years old, unmarried, divorced, currently employed at a seedy printing shop, car falling apart, renting, daughter won't speak to her. Son gone out to California somewhere.

Betty had lots of things to complain about and lots of things to worry about. She got married too young, she didn't like her work, she didn't like where she lived. The list was complete. The drinking had to stop. It hadn't helped. It had made things worse.

She would drink when she was feeling unhappy and she had fully expected for it to make her happy. She recalled when she was growing up seeing the ads on the television. She heard them on the radio. She saw them in the newspapers. They weren't in those vehicles too much anymore but the movies and songs were heavy laden with them. The people in the movies, for example, she noticed when they went out to dinner it always seemed to be a place that had a bar in the background. In the background, at least, sometimes they met in a bar or ate at a bar. It made her crazy.

What was even crazier was when she realized the week before when she was at a movie with her then-boyfriend, that they were serving liquor in the movie theater. You couldn't get away from it. All the magazines she read were peppered with ads for alcohol. It was crazy.

Her eyes were really opened up earlier in the week when she went looking for help. She stumbled across something called the 'Alcoholic Beverage Corporation'. It turned out it was some sort of government, state-run business or somehow controlled by the state government that was responsible for every single drop of alcohol in the state.

They determined prices, availability, territories for the companies making and distributing it. Yet, at the same time they were supposed to be helping people with their health. They were supposed to be protecting everyone from drunk drivers. That was a crock! She had been arrested the year before on a drunk driving charge. She had been able to 'plea it down' and get away with a big fat fine. There were about thirty or forty people in court the day she was there for the same thing. They pretty much all got the same thing she noticed. At least those she had seen. She had left after her case and the room was still full.

One guy there had been caught four times. They were going to put him in jail but the lawyers and the judge met together and the next thing you know he's walking out too!

Now she finds out they run the game. What is she supposed to do? Just go along with it?

She felt used before now she felt like a jerk.

She looked back at the computer screen. It was sitting frozen in its present state. Waiting for her to do something. To talk to someone.

They had all told her to talk to someone. The police, the lawyer, her daughter, her son, her ex-husband, before he disappeared when the kids were small. Just nuts!

She used to try and drink to get happy but it didn't work. It just made her unhappy.

When she was angry she had a few drinks to take the edge off. That didn't work either. It ended up just making her angrier. Some people called her an 'angry drunk'. She didn't think she was one. She couldn't remember any angry episodes but she had to admit drinking didn't make her feel less angry it often enraged her.

She used to feel that everyone her age drank excessively. Maybe she just had a problem. If she could solve the problem she could drink excessively and enjoy it too. Of course that was all a lie. Just a trick of her own mind fashioned out of the desires she had coupled with the advertisements and the lies in general.

She was embarrassed to speak to her peers. Embarassed to speak to anyone about it for so long, but now, today, tonight.

What would it change?

She thought about it.

'My life, for one.', she thought.

She clicked the mouse button to 'Send' the post and she sat and waited.

At first there were just one or two responses. 'Hang in there', 'You go, girl', and then there were others, 'I felt the same way', 'Let me tell you my story', 'This the way it was for me, you can do it too!', suddenly, there in this public forum were all these strangers giving her much needed advice, commiserating with her and attempting to help her.

She was caught unaware. What had started with one or two messages started turnining into a roaring torrent of interest, care and one or two smart-alecks. 'What did you think it would get you?' 'Straighten up and fly right'.

Then came the resources – who to call, what to do.

Betty had to stand up. She had to take a break.

She looked out the window. She knew she was going to be able to do it.

She looked back at the computer and began to cry.

'Why did I believe all those things? Where did those ideas come from?'

She started to feel like she needed a drink but she didn't get one. She sat down and started to read. She wrote back to a few people and then ended up printing everything they had sent so she could go through them and learn and act.

She called her daughter later than night.

'Hi Laura, this is your Mom calling.'

'Hi Mom, what do you want?', Laura asked.

'I just wanted to call and say hello. I'll call you again next week.'

The line was quiet.

'Laura?', Betty asked.

The pause continued.

Betty's heart skipped a beat in consternation. 'I should've known better.', Betty thought.

Laura's voice came over the line, 'Okay, Mom, I'll be looking forward to hearing from you next week.'

Betty said, 'Okay, bye now.'

Story 9

Anna

Anna had met Mike when she went to a Rehab Center in Illinois. It was her first time in a Rehab Center. It was Mike's third. He had been offered a plea deal where he could go and get help this one last time or he would go to jail for holding with intent to distribute.

Mike didn't really have the intention of getting away from the drug culture. He just wanted to get away from the prosecutor so he took the deal as soon as it was offered.

When in Rehab he had met Anna. He had some affection for her but what he felt for her could not be described as love. Anna had feelings for Mike and associated their physical contact with emotional contact. She was not able to see through the fog that Mike expressed in his life. She believed he had been lucky in getting the plea deal and thought he was on the road to recovery.

She believed that because he had been in Rehab before that he was experienced and could help her. The things he taught her how to do had very little to do with recovering from drug addiction.

One of her counselors had attempted to warn Anna but Anna was convinced she was helping Mike. It is possible that if Mike had not entered Anna's life that her time in Rehab might have been much shorter. As it was she got access to drugs once while in Rehab. Mike was the go-between. He only did this once because shortly after this episode he was kicked out of the center. He was immediately arrested and placed in jail for a six month term. During his time in the prison he was able to secure access to opioids from time to time.

As for Anna she completed her treatment. When she left the facility her father sent her to Alabama to live with relatives. When Mike got out of jail Anna spent her money and provided him with airline tickets to join her in Alabama. She thought that if the Rehab had not done the job on Mike then the jail time had. She was unaware that Mike had been in and out of jail for most of his life. He was not honest to her and concealed his past from her, both good and bad.

During this time Anna interacted with Mike's sister, Susan, who lived a distance away. She had three children that she lost custody of in Illinois. She was pregnant with a fourth child. She had lost custody because she was a repeat drug offender. She was an active heroin addict at the time she was interacting with Anna. She didn't reveal this until about a year after Anna had met her over a phone conversation.

Anna claimed to have kicked the habit a long time ago.

During the later part of the year Susan told Anna that her boyfriend had been abusive to her. He had beat her and stolen from her. Their relationship, to put mildly, was tumultuous. Local law enforcement and social workers were generally convinced that eventually either Susan or her boyfriend would end up dead and that not long in the future.

Susan asked Anna for help. She told Anna that all the shelters were full and she couldn't find any help from her family or friends. She claimed to be afraid of her boyfriend but also wanted to know if Anna could help the both of them. Anna didn't know what to do. She had limited resources. Her family had stopped talking to her again because it became clear that even though Anna had seemingly distanced herself directly from the drug culture that Mike, the man she had transported to her small town in Alabama from Illinois was an active drug addict. They believed that eventually he would draw her back into that life. They were filled with sorrow and remorse for helping her. They felt she had betrayed them.

She tried to tell Susan that there were other resources she could reach out for. She gave her all the information she had on the subject. It was like talking to a brick wall. Susan claimed that the resources that Anna was directing her to did not exist. In her own way Susan was abusing Anna. What Anna wasn't aware of was, that like her brother Mike, Susan wasn't telling Anna everything.

Susan was an active, pregnant drug user, that was correct. She was not, however, seeking any sort of assistance. She was waiting in fear and dread but also in longing for her boyfriend to get out of jail. She also didn't tell Anna that the baby she was currently carrying wasn't the result of her relationship with her boyfriend. When he found out anything could happen including deadly violence.

Still, Susan, in her addled state of mind believed that everything was fine. She represented this to Anna. What's worse is that Susan represented these affairs to anyone who would listen to her. She lied to a great body of people over and over again. Some of them, unlike Anna, actually sent her money. They pitied her, they believed, and gave her money which she used immediately to buy the drugs that poisoned her body, mind and soul and was ravaging the frail life attempting to begin within her womb.

Anna didn't know what to do or where to turn.

She didn't have the money or resources to help Susan.

The only thing that saved Anna was that Mike, who had taken up the practice of coming and going as he pleased without telling anyone, had gotten involved in petty crime. He was shot and killed during a robbery.

Anna was heartbroken. She convinced her parents to lend her money to bring Susan to Alabama to attend the funeral. She tried to contact Susan but Susan's husband had gotten out of jail. He moved the both of them California and Anna never heard from Susan again.

Brenda sat on the opposite side of the desk. She was holding her purse on her lap. Her hands were clenched and tight on the purse strap.

Ron sat facing her. His computer monitor was off to his right.

Ron said, 'How can I help you today?'

Brenda looked at him. She had arrived in the office about twenty minutes earlier. She had to sign in at the front desk and then wait until one of the social workers could talk to her. The greeter at the front was careful to tell her she might not be able to see anyone right away without an appointment.

It turned, out, however, that Ron's 1 o'clock appointment hadn't shown up. The man was a newly diagnosed addict who hadn't yet made the actual final decision to get away from drugs and the drug life. Ron saw many like him. He knew the young man would either decide to move on from it or be consumed by it. There was nothing he could do if the guy didn't show up for his appointments.

Brenda said, 'I'm visiting you to talk about a friend and ask some advice. Her family doesn't know what is going on and she doesn't want them to find out. She'd probably be here herself if she could but she can't.'

Ron said, 'There's very little I can do if the person doesn't present themself.'

'I was hoping you could give me advice.'

'Okay, let's see what we can do.'

Brenda continued, 'My friend has an opiate problem. Hydromorphone, I believe. Can't be sure. It could be morphine – I can't quite remember.'

Ron said, 'That's okay. We'll just go with opioid and he wrote on his pad.'

'She is trying very hard to come of the drugs. I know this because she told me.'

'I admire your confidence.'

'She's scared to stop because she knows how sick I got when I kicked the habit.' She laughed nervously. 'Okay, so, I was very sick but I don't think I handled it properly. I think I gave her a bad impression about the benefits of getting off the drugs.'

'As you know,', Ron spoke, 'it's different for everyone. Everyone has different experiences. It's not that yours was good or bad or that you provided a good or bad example – what you did was great! It's great for you and everyone you know. I hope you know that, Brenda.'

'Thank you. Are you a doctor?'

'Of sorts. I studied Social Work. Please continue.'

'What I would like to know is what I could to help her with her withdrawals? Is there anything I can do? She doesn't want to use pills no more. She wants to have a baby. She wants to be away from drugs for a year before she starts trying to get pregnant with her husband. Do you have any suggestions?'

'Well, this is all a big deal, Brenda. You're quite a friend to do what you are doing. I suggest your urge your friend to get some professional help. There are medications that will help her with withdrawals. I can give you some pamphlets on each one. There are two doctors in the area that specialize with working with mothers who are addicted to drugs or had been addicted in the past. They are close by and I can give you references to them. How are you doing, Brenda? Do you need anything?'

'Not right now, thank you. I am happy to help my friend out the worst kind of life I had. That's all. I don't want to have what I had. I don't want anyone to go through what I went through. I want her to have her baby and be happy with her family. She deserves that, you know?'

'Yes, I know. I also know that families can be hard. It's hard to get approval or forgiveness or whatever but family can be a very important part of anyone healing. Talking is always best but it depends on the circumstances. That's why I encourage your friend to come and talk. Sometimes a psychiatrist or psychologist can help ease the mental anguish that can come along with any physical pain from withdrawal. Also – after the drugs go away sometimes other things show up. Other problems that can be dealt with without the drugs.'

'What do you mean by that?'

'Some people get into drugs in the first place, Brenda, because they were sick or sick of something. They made the wrong moves or went through the wrong circumstances and ended up with a drug problem. Once they battle their way out of that they may come back to the problem they were trying to escape. That's where all the help they can get can come in handy.'

'I see what you mean.'

'Well, here are the contact sheets I can provide you. I can't give you any specific recommendations because I haven't met the woman and that would not be right. The things I tell you could be wrong. It would be best for her to stop in. We aren't going to tell her family or anyone anything she tells us. It's all private.'

'I'll do that. Thank you so much for all this. I really appreciate it. Thank you.'

'You're welcome.' Ron walked the young woman out to the front and waved good-bye.

He turned to go back to his office when the greeter called to him and said, 'Dr. Reynolds, your 1 o'clock just showed up. He wants to know if he can see you.'

Ron turned around and smiled.

'Yes, that will be fine.', he said.

'This is turning out to be a great day after all!', he thought and went to greet his client.

Story 11

Esmerelda

Esmerelda sat across from Patrick and looked at him with tearing eyes.

This was Patrick's first case on his own. He had set up everything as perfectly as he could imagine. He had an appointment made. His client, potential client, that is, actually showed up. If only he had a secretary it would have been fantastic! Oh, well, one thing at a time. He offered Esmerelda some coffee.

At first she demurred but then, seeming to consider it further, asked for a cup of coffee.

Patrick, how had just settled down into his leather chair worked himself back out of the seat and crossed the room behind Esmerelda to the small table that held the coffee pot, cups and condiments.

'Cream and sugar?'

'No, thank you.', came the answer.

Just as Patrick began back across the room Esmerelda's voice came again, 'Well, just one sugar a shot of cream if you don't mind.'

Patrick spun on his heel and went back to the coffee pot. He put the cup down a little too quickly and the coffee splashed out and gave him a little burn on his hand.

'Ooowee!', he whistled.

'Are you okay?', Esmerelda asked.

'Yes, yes, I'm fine.'

Patrick dried his hands, made a cup of coffee for Esmerelda and one for himself and returned to the desk.

He placed Esmerelda's coffee down in front of her and walked around to his chair. He sat down.

Esmerelda asked, 'Where should I begin?'

'Well, you can tell me why you've come to see me.'

'How much will this cost?'

'Well, at this point it is a consultation so it is free. We will discuss your case and you can decide, then how you would like to proceed with the firm.'

'Is it just you here right now?'

Patrick took a sip of his steaming coffee and winced as the hot liquid touched his upper lip. He shook his head quickly up and down, 'Yes, yes, I'm the one. This is my practice. Patrick Glenn.'

'Okay. Well, I'm getting kicked out of my apartment.'

'What did you do?'

'I was a week late on the rent.'

'Oh, well, a week? Is that all?'

'That's all I can see. I had some trouble with a job. I let the landlord know the problem and that I would pay. He said it would be okay but then he sent me an eviction notice three days later.'

'Well, did you agree to this sort of relationship at any point – that he might terminate the agreement at any time?'

'I don't think so. I just signed the normal paperwork for the lease. I don't think I agreed to getting kicked out whenever the landlord felt like it. My grandmother tells me I have all sorts of rights but I don't know what they are. Can you help me?'

'I can help you understand some of it. Essentially, depending on how much trouble you want for yourself you can act according to the eviction notice and move out or you can find out why he is trying to kick you out and fix that and see if your landlord still wishes to go through with the tenant eviction procedures or you could sit tight and the landlord will need to bring suit against you. If you choose the last then you will need some legal assistance.'

'Well, I don't have much money. In fact, I've got just enough to live on. You see, I've been a drug addict. I was using heroin quite a bit. I ended up going to a Rehabilitation Center. My parents paid a lot of money to make that happen. I got better, you see? I am eight months away from that place. I got a job a pizza parlor and was doing okay. I was able to get the apartment. Then, I got an offer from a gas station and went to work there – but the job didn't last. The owner let some guy that had left come back and I got the boot! I was short the rent and then the rest happened and I'm here to see you.'

'Well, you certainly are working hard. I can see that by what you've told me. Why didn't you ask your parents for money?'

'I was too embarrassed to ask them. I explained to the landlord I just needed one more week. Then he called me and told me someone had told him I was a drug addict and he wanted me out.'

'Did anyone hear him say that to you?'

'No, it was over the phone.'

'Well, that was wrong but there's not much to be done unless someone else could corroborate your story. We may be able to talk to him and see if something can be worked out. You shouldn't have to move. It must be hard what you're doing.'

'Will you help me?'

Patrick placed his elbows on his chair arms, he slowly brought his forefingers together in a point just under his upper lip, he thought to himself, 'I've always wanted to do that!'

Patrick said, 'Yes, I'll take the case.'

'How much will you charge me?'

Patrick said, 'This is my first case. I am waiving my fee. This will be done Pro Bono.'

'What's that?'

'For free, Miss Esmerelda, for free.'

She began to cry.

Story 12

Caroline and Her Mother

Caroline looked out the window at the driving snow.

There wasn't much she could do. She was at her wits end. Her mother had tried to help along the way and she had tried to help her mother. They had found housing in a small apartment complex in a quiet neighborhood. They kept to themselves and didn't bother anyone. They had made friends with some of their neighbors. They were very happy to know the young couple that lived across from them. They just had a new baby.

The year prior, however, things had begun to change. The family that had lived below them moved out. The apartment was empty for about a month when a new tenant moved in. Everything was quiet at first. In fact, it was very quiet, it was almost like no one was living there at all. No one ever saw the tenant and there didn't seem to be anyone coming and going. Sometimes early in the morning Caroline thought she heard noises from downstairs but chalked them up to the building settling or the wind.

Things changed after that first, month, however. There was lots more activity down below almost right away. The tenants sounded happy and boisterous. Late in the evening they would depart so everyone thought they worked nights. They would return in the late morning and things would be quiet until late afternoon when it start again.

The amount of quiet time, however, began to be reduced over time. Within two months it was apparent something strange was going on. Caroline had noticed a young man with reddish hair that seemed to be around most of the time but the rest of the traffic seemed to be random. You never knew who would show up. Timing was strange as well. There would be two days of no noise and a week or so of frenetic activity only to see it die down again.

The neighbors across the way became concerned. Especially since the woman had gotten pregnant. They didn't have it easy and had no quick way to get out of there, just like Caroline and her mother. Her other neighbors were composed of elderly people and a couple of single mothers. There were small families in the building across the way.

They neighborhood the buildings were located at was nice. It was middle class. Most of the homes were occupied and those that were not were for sale. There was a grocery store and other stores within walking distance.

There was a park down the block and Caroline and her mother would walk there when then weather was warm. Recently, however, Caroline didn't go out much at all. You never knew what was going on in the hall.

She had begun to notice people coming to the apartment below in cars. There would be loud blaring music from the speakers. Someone would jump out of the car, enter the building, enter the apartment below and come out shortly after. The man across the hall told Caroline he had seen people exchanging money and small packages at the door. He was pretty sure they were dealing drugs.

Caroline had come to the same conclusion herself. She had seen the same things her neighbor had. She had also seen others in the stairwell selling things to each other. She had even seen some of the people that came to the apartment building sit down on the steps and stick needles in their arms.

Whoever lived downstairs had dropped a bag of used needles on their way to the garbage container out back. Caroline just didn't know what to do.

Carolina had went to the landlord and even written to the property owners. At first the maintenance and management folks at the front office were supportive. They did what they could do. Caroline had heard and seen them threatened, however, and their ardor cooled after that. Caroline called the local police department. They had been responsive at first but a few times they had shown up and the offending car or people had left the area. They started to treat Caroline and her mother like they were the problem.

Sometimes they would show up and sometimes they would not. Other times they would show up hours later and come to bang on Caroline's door and never approach the door downstairs.

The young man with red hair became somewhat of a fixture in the area. He might be seen in the hallway below, or in the parking lot. During the warmer weather he stationed himself near the pool. The management had to close the pool eventually the last summer because of the people the young man was attracting to the area. They had also found a needle on the pool deck and one in the water. The mother who had found the needle on the pool deck made a big deal about it with the management company and they gave her another, larger apartment in another complex they owned across town.

As time went on and autumn ended winter started up. The activity became confined more and more to the first floor lobby area outside the apartment and in the apartment itself. The door was sometimes left open or just a little ajar. It was never vacant anymore. There was always some activity and the young man with red hair would appear regularly.

Sometimes the activity spilled onto the second floor landing. Caroline would get very upset at that time. At one point she thought a fight in the hallway was going to spill into their apartment and she would have two brawling addicts on her carpet in the living room.

One time an ambulance arrived and carried someone out from the first floor area. The apartment had been quiet for two days after that.

On that Friday, however, there was yelling. It appeared like there was going to be a fight. During the night over that weekend the yells and cries were from someone calling for money they were owed by whoever was in the apartment. Someone else called the police that evening but only after it sounded like several shots were fired.

When the police arrived they did find bullet holes in the glass of the sliding door of the apartment on the first floor. The man with the red hair told them, however, that he had been out at the time and hadn't seen who had done it.

The police departed.

Within a few hours there was what sounded like a full blown party below them.

Caroline eventually requested to be moved to another location. She was told she could go but because of the financial arrangement for her mother she would need to stay in the place for another year before she could move.

Caroline loved her mother and decided to stick it out. By the time they left the apartment complex a year later two people had died in the stairwell and another in the apartment below them.

About four months prior to their moving date the red hair man seemed to disappear. He wasn't seen around anymore. The apartment, though, remained as it was and had become. The loud gatherings continued without letup. The police left the place alone – their logic being that if they chased them out they would just go somewhere else.

Caroline and her mother were very happy when they moved into their new place.

The couple across from them moved away shortly after their baby was born. The husband said it would be better for him to struggle than to live near that.

Story 13

Darla and Happiness

Darla had been addicted to heroin for two years. She desperately wanted to stop using heroin.

She was able to enroll in a Rehabilitation Program that helped her out quite a bit. She was able to escape the clutches of her addiction and managed her body's cravings by taking Suboxone.

Suboxone is a drug that contains a combination of buprenorphine and naloxone. Buprenorphine is an opioid medication and referred to as a narcotic. Naloxone blocks the effects of opioid medication, including pain relief or feelings of well-being that can lead to opioid abuse. Suboxone is used to treat opioid addiction.

She and her husband decided to have a baby. Darla read everything she could find about having a baby while taking Suboxone. One of her doctors scared her quite a bit and she wasn't sure what would happen. As it was she met this doctor three months after she had discovered she was pregnant. Darla was miserable for a whole month.

Then she met another doctor who specialized in pregnancies for mothers that were actively addicted or were in treatment like Darla. Darla was fortunate to meet this doctor and learn what could be done to protect her own health and the health of her baby.

Darla went to see this doctor, Doctor Gilette, all through her pregnancy. He delivered the baby too and was there to check the baby for any signs of Neonatal Abstinence Syndrome. Neonatal abstinence syndrome (NAS) are a set of difficulties that happen in a newborn who was exposed to addictive opiate drugs while in the mother's belly.

Darlas was concerned about her baby because opioids and other substances pass through the placenta that connects the baby to its mother. The baby also becomes dependent on the drug along with the mother.

To make matters worse if the mother continues to use the drugs within the week or so before delivery, the baby will be addicted when born. Because the baby is cut off from the drug at birth they may experience withdrawal symptoms as the drug is slowly cleared from the baby's system. In some opioid cases the child may appear normal and sicken and die with a short time – from a few days to a week after birth.

Darla was also horrified to learn that withdrawal symptoms also may occur in babies exposed to alcohol, benzodiazepines, barbiturates, and certain antidepressants (SSRIs) while waiting to be born.

She became aware that in general babies of mothers who use other addictive drugs (nicotine, amphetamines, cocaine, marijuana,) may have long-term health problems.

In Darla's case the baby was born normally and did not experience the Neonatal Abstinence Syndrome. Darla was so happy about the baby and her health and the baby's health that she started to tell other people about it.

She was met with various responses. Her parents were critical pointing out that if she hadn't started using drugs in the first place she wouldn't have felt the need to feel relieved. That just didn't make sense to Darla so she let it pass. Many of her friends could not understand as they had not gone through what Darla had gone through when she stumbled into the disease of addiction. She was just glad to have them as friends even if they didn't understand that part of her life.

She was more concerned about the reaction of people she had come to know through the Rehabilitation Program and other drug-free circles she travelled in. Many of them were mean spirited and told her she had done wrong by putting the baby at risk. When she told her about what her experience doctor had said they unfairly called him a quack.

Others were convinced that she had been extremely lucky and anyone dealing with Suboxone during pregnancy was just plain crazy. Again – these people did not believe what Darla said herself and did not believe what the doctor said. They wouldn't even look at the literature she had on it – and it wasn't much.

She decided to make a video to share. She was very afraid because she expected that people would have negative things to say and attack her. When she offered up the idea in social media that's exactly what some people did.

About a year later Darla was on the verge of deciding against the video idea when someone she didn't even know contacted her and told her she was so glad that Darla had talked about her experience. This other woman told Darla that she had gone on through with her pregnancy because she had hope and was convinced she was doing the best thing for the baby by also following through Suboxone.

She had given birth to a healthy baby girl and was very happy.

Darla made her video and shared it. She believed that is she could help someone feel better about themself and their unborn child she would have done good. She felt it was right to help them become educated in their situation and let them lead themselves to happiness.

Story 14

Wanda and The Preacher

The preacher looked at Wanda.

The room was small. It was lined with wood paneling. There was a printer machine in the corner with a FAX machine attached to it. There were two small book cabinets. One was filled with the books the preacher had brought – the included pamphleteers, Bibles, notebooks, collections of sermons and items sent from the main office. The other book case was a hodgepodge of books left over from the previous preacher. They included much of the same that Reverend James kept and was supplemented with Bible Stories for Children, cookbooks and hymnals. Reverend James had taken the habit of removing one or two books per week and placing them in the small library in the common room.

He was looking at how many he had left to do as Wanda was talking.

On his desk was an invitation to some sort of meeting held by or for addicts – that is, those who were suffering from addiction as the flyer said. He received invitations like this from time to time. He was relatively sure he would have to skip this one as well. His duties at the church usually left him with precious little time for any work in the community.

Wanda was a slim woman. In her early 40's. She had been a long time church member. She attended most all of the Sunday services and showed up about once a month for the services and prayer meetings on Wednesdays. She contributed to the church regularly though she wasn't one of the heavy hitters.

Reverend James looked at her and made a conscious effort to concentrate.

'What brings you here to see me, today, Wanda? How's that daughter of yours?'

Wanda's face dropped considerably. It looked like she was going to cry for a moment. She sobbed and drew in her breath sharply. She said, 'That's what I've come to talk to you about.'

'I want to tell you what happened.'

'Oh, my. Take your time, then.'

He had seen he had misttepped. This had been happening to him too frequently lately. He had to improve his concentration. He was beginning to feel he was out of step with the needs of those around him. It wasn't a crisis of faith, just a realization that he needed to adjust some things. He just didn't know what.'

Wanda continued, 'I want to speak to you about my recent experiences. It's about this epidemic...'

Reverend James looked confused for a moment, he was really getting blindsided, 'Uh, excuse me, Wanda, what epidemic?'

'The opioid epidemic, Reverend James. That's what it's called. So many young people, so many people of all ages are caught up in it. Some of them are dying.'

She did start to cry at this time. Reverend James offered her a tissue. She took it and dried her eyes and blew her nose.

'It's a sickness. A sickness. This epidemic, this addiction devastated myself and my family. Erin is dead. She died two days ago. This is the first time I am out. I want to ask you to officiate at the funeral.'

'Yes, yes, of course, we'll make all the arrangements for you. I'll have Judy take care of it.'

Judy was the church administrator.

Wanda went on, 'I was afraid couldn't tell you this without crying my eyes out. I prayed and prayed on it and came to the conclusion that it is more important to share what happened to me than keep it to myself. I can't imagine anyone else going through this. I am having trouble believing it is happening to me. She was in college, she just got a new car, she had a very nice boyfriend and now, two days later all that is in the past. I just don't understand it.'

She cried again.

Reverend James said, 'Take your time.' He sat back and waited.

Wanda spoke, 'She fought with addiction for at least three years. That what I know for sure. There may have been other things when she was younger but I must have missed it. It doesn't matter now. These things come on so fast. It's insane!

It turns out that she was addicted to just one thing either. She was into two or three things she had to have all the time. Heroin or opioid pills, mood relaxers, they call them benzodiazepines and alcohol. It was horribly amazing. I had no idea. How can you function when all that is in your system and yet she did!

About two months ago I found out that people who are addicted are often caught up in more than one drug. So much has happened in the last two months, it's just a whirlwind!

You know, she had a son who just turned five. He's been with me. He's going to stay with me. He's just realizing she's not coming back. She's with my sister right now. He's been through a lot on his own. I knew she had problems but she was good at hiding them. I am just glad he is alive. He's had it very hard.

I've never dealt with this kind of situation before. I don't know what to do at this time. People don't want to talk about it. Along with her I know of three other people that have died from overdose s in the past year. Bill McKinney, the McKinney's boy, he died from it.'

The pastor said, 'I thought that was a heart attack.'

Wanda looked stricken, 'Oh, maybe I shouldn't have said that, but everyone is so quiet and this monster is wandering around out there and no one wants to speak its name. He died of a heart attack but he had been using drugs for some time. It destroyed his life. It killed him.'

'I wasn't aware of that. I thought he had some congenital heart disease.'

'Whether it was congenital heart disease or the disease of addiction, it doesn't matter, together they killed him. All the horror and sorrow before and Mrs. McKinney told me about it and now Eriin's gone! I can't bear it!'

She cried quietly for a minute and continued, 'I lost my daughter. I want you to know I'm no expert in addiction. I'm not an ex-addict. I'm not a psychiatrist or some fancy addiction doctor. I tried to help her. I did my best. I'm so confused. I helped her, I thought I did, when I think back on it and see all that was going on I wonder if I was putting too much pressure on her. Did I do this to her? I just don't know. I don't want it to be. I want it to be over and her to come home.'

Wanda held her head in her hands and then sat back up.

I tried to show her a mother's love. The love of God. I thought she knew but she left anyway. She died anyway.'

Reverend James sat in rapt attention. His mask of godliness stripped away in the face of this raw information.

'I wanted to help and it turns out she was manipulating me and lying to me in so many ways. I love her so much and I am so angry with her. So angry for her treating me with the way she did, but more than that, angry with how she treated her son, how she treated herself. Didn't I raise her right? What did I do wrong?'

Oh, it's so much!

You wouldn't believe, Reverend, how many people told me not to worry. Just let her 'hit bottom'. What is that, Reverend? What's bottom? People say they get high and to get them to stop they have to hit bottom? What are these ideas? Where did they come from? They don't make sense!

Towards the end I would tell them, 'You know what's at the bottom? Death! Death is at the bottom!'. I thought she had stopped. I really did. Now my grandson is with my sister and I have to get him later. What do I need to do about these arrangements?'

The sudden change of the conversation took Reverend James by surprise. He responded, 'I'll have Judy contact you this afternoon. Just give me the contact information for you…and your sister, if that's okay.'

'That's okay.'

Wanda went through her bag and began writing out the information on a pad and pen she produced. She went on talking, 'I did a lot of things to protect her that might be considered shameful. I made a lot of mistakes. Now I'm left to clean up the mess. I'm left behind. I feel so guilty. Her lost to me, it's so gargantuan. So large. So huge.'

She handed the slip of paper over to the Reverend and said, 'Thank you.'

Wanda left.

Reverend James sat for a minute collecting his thoughts. His eyes roved around the room and came to rest on the flyer on his desk. He called Judy into his office and explained the situation with Wanda and her daughter and what needed to be done. When Judy left Reverend James picked up the phone and called the number on the flyer.

When a voice answered at the other side he said, 'Hello, my name is Reverend James. I am calling to see if you need a place to hold meetings. I would like to come to the next one if I could.'

Story 15

Miranda

Miranda was looking unhappy.

She had been happy for a while, she told me. She and her husband had parted ways after the children grew up. She remained in the town they had settled in and he had moved on to the other side of town.

He had been drinking for a long time. Since he was a teenager and had taken up drugs shortly thereafter. He went from job to job until he found a steady position working nights in a warehouse. The money was not too bad and with Miranda working at the same time they were able to raise a family together.

They had a boy and a girl. Both of them did well though they had to grow up in a house that was always teetering in disaster. Miranda's husband Vic would sometimes drink himself into a stupor and at other times launch into vitriol and loud language. He was abusive to Miranda and eventually she could take no more and divorced him. He had very little contact with the children even before the divorce so they didn't miss him much.

Miranda guided them through school and they both went on to college and were attending in a town near where they had grown up.

In August of the previous year Miranda and both children had received word from his side of the family that Vic was in the hospital and in danger of dying. He had experience complete liver failure. The two children made their way to their father and Miranda went along as well so that the children would not be alone in that situation. The medical situation worsened over the course of a day and the doctors didn't expect Vic to pull through but pull through he did.

As Miranda told me his side of the family had very little to do with Vic. They didn't support him and it was amazing that they had called her from the hospital. His sister had gone to see him when he called her. Vic's sister had left the hospital directly after phoning Miranda and the children and had not returned.

Miranda's children were relieved their father was okay and went on with their lives and started college in the fall.

Through a strange set of circumstances that involved incomplete forms, conversations and incidents Miranda had begun to take on the role of caretaker for Vic. He wasn't as abusive as he once was and directed most of his ire towards other but the faint hint of aggression towards Miranda always hung in the air.

She did what she could for Vic. She went to the market for him. Picked up his medications. Filled out forms for him and did other things. At first she was comfortable with the situation thinking that it would not last long but as it progressed she got the feeling that Vic expected this to continue far into the future.

Miranda didn't know what to do about it until one day she had brought some groceries over to Vic's house and found beer in the refrigerator. She was struck by the enormity of what he had done and what she had been doing.

'He was dying!', she told me.

She couldn't believe he would go out and get the very poison that had put him in the hospital and nearly killed him. She told me that she knew it was a disease but still hadn't perceived that maybe the disease had made her sick too.

Made her sick to his lies and deceit.

She went, after she had seen the beers, to his medicine cabinet. He sat sitting in front of the television watching some sports program with glassy eyed intent. She opened the glass on the mirrored cabinet and found among the personal items stored there a container of oxycontin pills.

Miranda told me she had told him that she would walk away from him if he drank.

Then she asked me what I thought she should do.

I prepared a pot of tea and asked her to explain the situation to me again. She repeated the material nearly verbatim but added in a couple of anecdotes where it was clear that the verbal abuse in the relationship had not stopped.

I asked her if the children had witnessed any of this and she told me they hadn't.

She repeated again how she told Vic she would leave if he started drinking again.

I said, 'Well, it looks like you found out he is drinking and taking drugs.'

She said, 'But he won't admit to it.'

I told her, 'He's probably not going to admit to it. Why would he push you away? He's got you where he wants you. You can see with your own eyes the evidence of what you told him would push you away but because he doesn't say it to you out loud you don't believe it.'

She was quiet for a moment.

She said, 'I can't watch him kill himself.'

I said, 'It's up to you, Miranda, but I believe you've done enough.'

'What more can I do?', she asked.

I said, 'The children need you, Miranda. Vic needs to take care of himself.'

Miranda and I had drank our tea and then she left. I spoke to her about a month later.

She told me she had helped Vic along for another week. She had gone over to his house to drop off groceries and one of his friends was there. They were both drinking and as high as kites.

She dropped off the groceries and hadn't gone back since.

She told me she was looking forward to her son graduating from college in two years. Her daughter would be following along a year after that.

Miranda was looking happy.

www.ingramcontent.com/pod-product-compliance
Lightning Source LLC
Chambersburg PA
CBHW051124250726
48655CB00007B/2865